I0426680

Stay Away From

Cancer

~daniscloset~

No food alone can protect you against cancer. A combination of healthy fruits and vegetables strengthens the immune system for better health. Strong evidence shows that a healthy planned diet, filled with lots of plant foods like blueberries, beets, whole grains, beans, cherries, avocado, rosemary, cinnamon, garlic, sweet potatoes, and so much more, can lower the risk.

An anti-cancer diet is a great way to reduce your risk of cancer. The ACS (American Cancer Society) says, "If you eat at least five servings of fruits and vegetables each day, with the right servings, you can stay healthier, even with little or no exercise".

This book will show you how to include some of the following foods and drinks in your diet: kumquat, raspberries, cranberries, pumpkin, cinnamon, garlic, mango, persimmon, tomato, lime, apples, strawberries, kiwi, lemon, lingonberry, currant, basil, ginger, onion, sage, sesame seeds, cloves, galangal, bell pepper, bok choy, turnip and mustard greens, zucchini, eggplant, fennel, baked fish, chicken (dark), salmon, half percent or skim milk, unsweetened tea, water, honey and lemon, carrots, apple juice (freshly squeezed), peanuts, pumpkin seeds, brown rice, black rice, oatmeal, cashews, natto, chestnut, and more.

Diet and Exercise

In case you're wondering how much a daily routine of diet and exercise affects your risk for cancer? Well, much more than you may think.

A poor diet and no activity are the two main factors that increase the risk of cancer. Staying at a healthy and manageable weight is the key.

Over eating infectious foods can cause obesity and problems to the breast tissue, rectum, colon, endometrial, pancreas and other parts of the body.

Foods that prevent cancer from occurring are generally the same. Fruits, veggies, and grains, they all have important nutrients for fighting substances like phyto-chemicals and pectin to strengthen the immune system. People who have a diet free of animal products, high in plant foods, and low in cholesterol has a much lower risk of developing this disease.

A lot of activity is needed to keep active and give energy to the body. It helps reduce your risk by helping with weight control, hormone levels, and the electrolyte system. Physically it helps with the reduction of heart disease, diabetes, and fatigue.

The Centers for Disease Control and Prevention (CDC) suggests that "Individuals should engage in moderate-intensity physical activity for at least 30 minutes on five or more days of the week, sedentary lifestyle were the most common cancers in the United States, (breast and colon cancer).

Most people work-out to prevent heart disease, but exercise can also play a key role in preventing cancer because the body is building up energy to help the immune system fight against germicides . Most cancers are caused by lifestyle factors not genes.

If you have this disease or undergoing treatment, it's important to take better care of yourself. The best ways to do this is to stay physically active. Certainly you don't want to wear yourself out, but in other words do something. It's wise to put in some form of exercise to your daily routine—primarily during therapy.

risk factors. Most of the studies suggest that people who eat more red meat have a higher risk for developing cancer than those who eat less red meat. For example, evidence from (ACS) states that "processed meats like hot dogs, bacon, and salami, increases the chances of colorectal cancer."

Many physicians are now founding that people can eat at least 18 oz of red meat a week without initiating the invitation to cancer. Choosing leaner cuts is more important selecting flank steak or extra lean ground beef.

Dairy:

Dairy is a varied food group, and it usually gives a good source of calcium. They are not good foods to fight off cancer, but if calcium levels are normal, it can help strengthen other parts of the body.

Types of Cancer

Breast Cancer:

Generally the first sign of breast cancer is a breast lump or an abnormal mammogram. It ranges from early curable breast cancer, to severe breast cancer, with a variety of breast cancer treatments. Male breast cancer is pretty much uncommon but must be taken seriously too. It forms in tissues of the breast which begins in the lining of the milk ducts, the narrow tubes that carry milk from the lobules of the breast to the nipple). Causing it to become invasive, - invasive is the type of cancer that has spreaded from where it began in the breast ducts circulating normal tissue. This can happen in both male and female breast, although the male's is quite rare.

When checking for breast cancer individuals are encourage to examine by stretching the arm over the back of the head, while using the forehand to palpate for lumps. If found, the growth will start to form a large grouping (tumor) that separates from cells, growing at a more rapid pace. This can invade surrounding tissue or spread to other parts of the body, known as metastasizing. Cells that metastasize can cause serious and fatal health complications when left untreated. The majority of breast cancer diagnoses occur in women, which is the second most common cancer diagnosis other than skin cancer in the U.S.

It is important to recognize symptoms early on, to increase the chances of effective treatment and survival as much as possible. Unfortunately, too many people primarily women, are not diagnosed early enough to undertake preventative treatments. On the other hand, regular mammograms ouch!!! And self examinations can help with chances of survival, if sought early on.

Colon Cancer:

It is caused by out-of-control cell growth. This uncontrollable cell growth initiates with cells in the large intestine. They are small benign tumors called adenomatous. This starts off as polyps that are on the inner lining of the large intestine. Many of them can grow into malignant colon cancers over time, if they are not removed during colonoscopy. Colon cancer cells will invade and damage healthy tissues that are near the tumor causing many complications.

After malignant tumors form, cancerous cells may start to travel through the blood stream and lymphatic system, spreading to other parts of the body. These cells can grow in several other places, invading and destroying other healthy tissues throughout the body. This process is called metastasis, and the result is a more serious condition that is very hard to treat.

Colon cancer is not the same as rectal cancer, but they do correlate together in what is called colorectal cancer. Rectal cancer circulates the rectum, which is the last part of the large intestine, near the anus. However, thanks to newer treatments early detection has saved over a million U.S. citizens.

Skin Cancer:

Skin cancer occurs when errors (mutations) occur in the DNA of skin cells. This causes cells to grow out of control forming layers of cancer cells.

Skin cancer begins in the top layer of the skin called the epidermis. The epidermis is a very narrow layer that provides a protective layer of skin cells that your body sheds on its own.

It is said that the two most common types of skin cancers are called basal cell and squamous cell cancer. They usually form on the hands, arms, face, and neck. Another type is called melanoma, this is more dangerous but less common. Every person is at risk for cancer, but it is more predestine for people who spend a lot of time in the sun like lighter skin tones, or over the age of fifty.

Too much exposure to the sunlight is the main reason for skin cancer. The sun contains ultraviolet (UV) rays and that alters the biological material in skin cells, causing mutations. Heated tanning salons, laser light machines, continuous X-rays, and sunlamps, can cause damage to the skin. People who work outdoor jobs meaning excessive sunbathing, (scorching sunbaths) poses a bigger risk. This may also include new freckles forming to the face or dark marks because of too much sunlight.

Cervical Cancer:

Has been identified as human papillomavirus (HPV) infection. This is usually caused by having multiple sex partners, long-term birth control pills, and engaging in early sexual contact. This is also known as cervical dysplasia or unusual growth in the cervical cells.

Many adults have been infected with a sexually transmitted disease at some point in their life. It may go away on its own, but sometimes it can cause genital warts or lead to cervical cancer. That's why it is so very important for women to have Pap tests and cancer screenings on a regular basis. A Pap test can identify changes in cervical cells before they transform into cancer. You should never be afraid of going to the doctor because you're scared of getting bad news. Treat this early on, you may prevent cervical cancer.

It is quite rare that a female will experience symptoms. But you may have symptoms if those cells change into cervical abnormality. Each cancer aforementioned are some of the main cancers that are becoming more and more common over time, but all of them will show similarity when cells are being destroyed.

Treatments

There are several different ways that a specialist can approach cancer for treatment, depending upon the circumstances, the type of cancer, and its current stage. These particular treatments are commonly used in the healthcare industry today; lasers, hypothermia, surgery, medications, chemotherapy, radiation and immunotherapy.

Laser Therapy:

Is a high volume of-intensifying light used for treatment and other diseases. Lasers can be used to shrink the size of a cancer tumor. It is most commonly used to treat superficial cancers that are on the surface of the body or the lining of internal organs. Such as, basal cell skin cancer, cervical, vaginal, and lung cancer.

For example, lasers can be used to shrink or destroy a tumor that is blocking a person's windpipe or esophagus. Also it can be used to remove colon polyps or tumors that are blocking the colon or stomach. On the other hand, the effects of laser surgery may not be permanent, so the surgery may have to be repeated more than once.

Hypothermia:

Deep tissue hyperthermia is used to reach tumors that are located deeply beneath the skin.

Prior to the procedure, a cat scan (CT) is done to specifically pinpoint the location.

A water-filled tube is placed on top of the individual's abdomen and electromagnetic energy is directed at the tumor, the tumor must be heated between 104°F to 107°F. This kind of treatment dilates blood vessels around the tumor, causing oxygen to carry red blood cells into the tumor.

If the patient is later on exposed to radiation treatment, it then reacts with the high levels of oxygen in the tumor, destroying the cells altogether.

If the person is getting chemotherapy, the blood flow to the tumor will bring more of the chemotherapy towards the tumor. Deep tissue hyperthermia can take up to two hours or more, and usually done twice a week for the duration of the chemo treatment. Most of its side effects are generally minimal.

Surgery:

Surgery is the removal of the tumor and surrounding tissue during an operation. A doctor who specializes in cancer surgery is called a surgical oncologist. Surgery is the oldest type of cancer therapy and remains as an affective treatment for all type of cancers today.

The choice of surgery varies. It is often used to remove all or some of the cancerous tissue after diagnosis. It can also be used to diagnose cancer, find out where the cancer is located, whether it has spreaded, and the affects to other organs.

The location where you have surgery depends on the duration of the surgery and how much recovery is needed. Surgery may be performed in a doctor's office, clinic, surgery center, or hospital.

Outpatient surgery means that you do not have to stay overnight in the hospital before or after it's done. Inpatient surgery means that you do need to stay in the hospital overnight or longer to recover from it.

Medications:

Medications have been around since the early days of cancer. The use has been limited due to lots of other reasons like medicine abuse and overdoses. This has changed in past years using current drugs like, cytotoxic, capecitabine, vinorelbine, and topotecan. These available oral agents are most effective for large tumors like ovarian, lung cancer, breast, and colon. Many prefer the oral way to cope with pain and stress without the side effects of I.V. needles and frequent hospital visits. Even at the expense of interference with clinical efficacy.

Chemotherapy:

Chemotherapy is a combination of powerful drugs to kill off cancer cells. Chemo can be used in addition with radiation or surgery to ensure that all cells will die off. Chemotherapy is administered in three different ways; intravenously, oral, and injections.

Intravenous: Is the most popular. A needle is placed into the vein while attaching its tubing to a plastic bag holding the drugs. The needle is removed at the end of each treatment. People who have several different chemotherapy sessions, generally has a plastic disc called a medic-port placed under the skin to work as an IV connection.

It is attached to a metal pole with flexible wheels providing convenience and mobility for the patient.

Others may be attached to a twenty four hour pain pump; this is usually given to patients who are in their fourth stage of cancer.

Oral chemotherapy: These are pills taken either by mouth or in a liquid format. As stated before, many will choose the route of oral to reject the idea of being poked with needles. Not everyone can stand the sight of a needle going into their veins; so oral meds will continue to serve a great purpose in today's world.

Injections: are vein punctured into the muscle underneath layers of skin or directly into a lesion. Whatever stage or type of cancer you may have will decipher how long you will receive your chemo.

You may get chemo treatments in either increment during the week or on a monthly schedule.

Once the body has become immune to the chemo and develops healthy new cells, then many doctors will consider giving a break between treatments.

Radiation:

Radiation therapy uses high frequency energized radiation to minimize tumors and kill off cancer cells. X-rays are said to be charged particles chosen for this particular type of treatment. It may be sent through a machine outside the body called external-beam radiation therapy, or either it comes from radioactive material administered into the body near the cells, called internal radiation therapy or brachytherapy. Just about every cancer patient will receive some type of radiation therapy during the course of his or her treatment.

Immunotherapy:

Immunotherapy is the kind of treatment that picks specific parts of a person's immune system to eliminate unhealthy cells. It is designed to trigger the body's natural defenses to start the movement of fighting away cancerous cells. The process starts by using the body's own immune system or laboratory methods to restore immune functions. However, all findings are not certain on how this treats the cancer but it has proven itself by slowing down the process and stopping a large number of cancer cells.

Success Stories

Mr. & Mrs. John Hernandez

Palm Beach, Florida

Mr. and Mrs. Hernandez grow a garden each summer to eat healthy, and save money on fruits and vegetables. Mr. Hernandez is the main caregiver who tends to the garden most of its time. He waters, pluck weeds, and make sure sunshine is not over exposed. This may sound easy but it certainly requires lots of time and effort.

Mr. Hernandez knows that if he stays away too long, or neglect the ability to care for his garden, he will not get a good outcome of fruits and vegetables.

After his big scare with polyps nearly two years ago, he changed his eating habits while reading "*Home Style Magazines*" to keep him informed on how others beat cancer when eating blueberries & wheat germ, and a dash of cinnamon each day. His persistence with the new diet even encouraged his wife to do the same. Both admitting that it was horrible starting off, but after a few weeks it got easier, and it was like introducing themselves to a new soft drink that has not hit the market yet.

Unlike their neighbors Savanna and Harold Peach, they could care less about eating healthy as well as believing in the myth of rarely cooked animals can do no harm to your body if kept fresh.

However, the Hernandez's still show great gratitude when it comes to supplying their neighbors with fresh foods. They deliver as often as they can baskets of sweet strawberries, crispy green bell peppers, banana cuts, and wheat sticks. Oppose to the sugary dinner rolls and chocolate pound cakes that are left near their door step from time to time, secretly donating it to their local church and the homeless who hangs around "Central Park".

It sure would be nice to have the Peach's join in with are new diet, "said Mrs. Hernandez." I over heard Francis and Mrs. Peach talking about her return visit from the doctor the other day, I didn't mean to ease drop but, they were just too loud in trying to cover it up. Do you think that I should say something in regards to how our health has change over the years, with the change in all? "I will leave that up to you my Dear, replied Mr. Hernandez. In the mean time I will be out in the garden. I need to make sure enough holes are punched into the ground. I hear the storm is coming. I don't want anything to flood over especially with my blueberries; somehow they just seem to energize me'.

Paul Salice

Owensboro, Kentucky

Paul Salice is a 35 year old male who is married with two small children. Paul works on the assembly line at "Koply Motors" Corporation. He was hired shortly after graduating from high school. He remains as a faithful Stuart who shows up everyday to work on time and maintains a positive relationship with all of his co-workers.

It only takes a split second to pick up the oily engine car parts, and throw them on the line for finish-up by his peers. Day in and day out, oil and grease is transferred from one station to another. This is the norm "Paul says'. We all have this in common, dirt is share among all of us here, but we understand this is our place of work.

Break room stations have no special treatments in this line of work. Everyone's evidence is shared among black oily fingerprints along the walls and staircases. Even the microwave that we use has not been prep for cleanliness in years. The secret we just buy new ones when they burn out.

The Responsibility comes with cleaning your own area here, but the truth is no one really does. We just create enough space for preparation until our thirty-minute break is up. I'm not sure if others wash their hands or not, I don't ask. Minding my own business is the safe way around this place.

During this time Mr. Salice is entering into his 17th year at "[Koply Motors]" Corporation. He has been promise an upcoming position as a new manager. This would be much more rewarding than standing up for eight hours examining heavy metal car parts.

He dreams of this position as a manager which would allow him very little contact with car parts and debris. Updating reports and sitting in meetings all day just seemed easier. *"I can almost taste it"* he said. This would even include a pay raise for him and his family and Paul's worries would be over.

According to Mr. Dudley, another manager, Paul was surely at the top of the list. He stopped by Paul's station each morning to reassure him of a job well done and how honored they are to consider him for the next candidate.

Paul could not help but to finally ask the big question. "When will I have my first interview with the owner"? He stated. "Timing is everything son" said Mr. Dudley, and you will be notified as soon as we hear something. His anticipation grew intensely, but this did not stop Paul from keeping his faith in the upcoming position as a manager.

As time moved on, Paul finally started to get emails from the owner and other managers in the company. His first email assignment was to give a brief description on how he would handle company affairs such as, tardiness, disputes among co-workers, productions rates, finances, privacy acts, weather hazards, and safety hazards. This would include a video of himself explaining each detail with printed documentation of each word announced. He really didn't know where to start, but Paul knew he had to do something. Besides, this was his only real shot to impress all the managers and its owner.

Paul began to search every possible website that could help him with tips on presentations and personal job descriptions. A good research would lead up to an extraordinary presentation.

A month had passed since Paul received his first email assignment, and the upcoming interview was near. Even though he was thrilled with excitement, and confident that he would get the position, he could not help but to feel an overwhelming of anxiety within himself. Paul knew that one mistake could cost him his future career as a manager with "Koply Motors".

The big day had finally come as Paul set in the conference room with Tom Brady (owner), Frank Dudley, and Samuel Castleberry two company managers. There was no time for last minute rehearsals or clearing his throat several times to get a good tone. So, Paul stood up in a quick array and stated, "Hello my name is Paul

Salice". I stand before you with plans and procedures for the next two years including financial budget plans and rules and regulations for this company.' Each person notice a big smile on each others faces because no one had ever planned projects two years in advance like this one.

At a great start Paul immediately begin to win favor because of his unique way of pre-advancing his ideas into the nearest future. All eyes gazed upon him, as he featured his presentation with his new fancy Apple Laser I pad. No one had ever seen a presentation done this way before. This way of performance had left much thought in the minds of all the conference participants and could not help but to wonder will he become the company's new manager.

Suddenly, the clock strikes twelve and Paul had to bring it to a close. Upon leaving his big performance he felt highly confident that he would make management real soon and all the worrying would be over.

After a long day of work Paul heads home to his wife and three children, running swiftly so eager to see them. He couldn't help but to take the first chair closest to the door. What's wrong Mrs. Salice ask Paul? Nothing more than usual Dear just a long day at work. But I must say I have been feeling a bit queasy lately, you mind getting me the pink stuff. Sure, as she started her way to the kitchen. She reached for the pink stuff and quietly yells, when was the last time you seen your doctor. I'm sure it's not that serious Dear just bring me the pink stuff and I will be fine. I know but I still think it would be a good idea to give Dr. Brown a call first thing in the morning. "FINE! I'll give a call", Paul replied.

The next morning was decision day, as Paul sat in the conference room with owner Tom Brady and head manager Frank Dudley. Why isn't anyone saying anything Paul thought to him self? It would be so much easier if they'd just come out and say it. Somehow the day just felt slow-motioned with a stomach full of knots. Couldn't they just speed up the process to stop the sweat from rolling down my armpit? I just want it to be over and finalized.

After a long discussion in the corner of the conference room, both men decided that Paul would be asked to give a last minute speech for clarity adding no inconsistency from his previous presentation. So he did. And once again Salice stood out; making a great impression that could never be forgotten. As he told the story of updating outdated machinery to newer technology, and the elimination of smoking areas for a healthier environment. The two gentlemen were so impressed that Brady suddenly blurts out Let the celebration began! There is nothing more to be said. Please call the secretary and tell her to order twelve large boxes of pizza, seven liters of soda, and one small order of spicy wings.

As time went on, Paul could not wait to slip away and phone his wife of the good news. Maybe she would come out and celebrate with him. This was the moment he had been waiting for, making bigger bucks and to land partnership of a brand new office and chair.

After prancing around a couple of hours in his new office, it was time to turn the lights down and head home. Coming home this particular day Paul noticed a very unusual look on his wife's face. What's wrong Dear, as he started out at her? Is it the kids, is everything okay. Yes Hun, the kids and I are fine but, I'm not so sure about you. What do you mean you're not so sure about me? Well, Dr. Brown call today, remember that visit I asked you to schedule. Yeah! Well, your test results are in. He wants you to get over to his office right away.

Paul grabbed the keys and rushed right over to Florida State Hospital barging through the door of Dr. Brown's office. "Hello Paul, said Dr. Brown, you're just the man I want to see have a seat in room two and I will be right with you.

Returning to room two, Dr. Brown began to go through Paul's chart. Paul immediately states; I sure hope it's not the "C"word, that disease is spreading all over. Dr. Brown had no intention of telling Paul right away that he indeed had cancer and it has spread, throughout his entire body. Also taking into consideration his wife had told Dr. Brown the good news about Paul's promotion earlier that day. Dr. Brown's response was very heart-broke and puzzling. "Let's just say a prayer first" Dr. Brown insisted.

After a quick word of prayer, Dr. Brown has chosen to give Paul a hint of the message. He said, "Well kid, if it is cancer than I want you to know that you are stronger than what you know. As for now, change your eating habits and wear all of your safety equipment at work. And we will talk about it more on Wednesday during your next visit. CHOW! Congrats on your new promotion.

Lillie Mae Peterson

Jackson, Mississippi

Lillie Mae Peterson is an 80 year widower who is known as one of the greatest cooks in Jackson Mississippi. She loves to invite all of her family and neighbors to her home for a delicious meal. Her biggest request is her sweet potato pies that she so loves to brown on top, with lots of butter.

For years Lillie Mae has kept the same recipes until her husband Freddie Peterson was diagnosed with cancer in {2002}. She was always certain that if she measured just the right amount of butter and lard it could do no harm to their cholesterol levels. However, getting educated with a new diet by Dr. Monsue, in [2003], she changed her cooking habits.

Dr. Monsue's dietary tips included a list of ingredients and levels of serving for all of his patients. His nutrition packet is usually sent home with every person showing exactly how to portion their foods, and what foods to choose for a good healthy meal. Lillie Mae has chosen to follow it!

After one year of following Dr. Monsue's food chart, Lillie begin loosing weight. She even felt a burst of energy out of no where, something she had never had before. This was a convincing "eye opener" for Mrs. Lillie, because she had always ate and cooked things just the way she liked it, without the interference of someone else.

Lillie Mae Peterson, Interview (2004)

Interviewer: Danielle McSpadden

Interviewee: Lillie Mae Peterson

Danielle: What are your favorites to cook?

Lillie Mae: *Well, my favorite thang to cook is my uh, sweet potato pies with a block of butter and I put dem in the oven so they can get brown on top. My next favorite is my collard greens with extra hog mogs and fat for better taste*

Danielle: Do you have health problems?

Lillie Mae: *Yup, I have diabetes and high blood pressure it runs in my family. But Dr. Monsue put me on a new diet and my sugar went down, so did my pressure.*

Danielle: What's the new diet?

Lillie Mae: *He told me I could keep my collard greens because they healthy for me. But not to put the mogs and fat in it. Because it raises my pressure. And for my sweet potato pies, take away the butter and put a little artificial sweetner in it and just oil the pans. And mo fruits & veggies.*

Danielle: Is this diet working for you?

Lillie Mae: *Yes Lord, its working. I never felt betta in a my whole life. I got mo energy now than when I was a teenager. But I still feel bad tho because I think I killed my husband. He didn't know how to cook he was just eat'n cause it was good. I always wondered if I had Dr. Monsue's diet stuff then, maybe he could of lived. But I'm still grateful* *to God that I didn't get cancer or nothing else, and*

still have a chance to live to see my great

grandbabies.

Danielle: Does your food still taste the
same? Does family and friends still come by?

Lillie Mae: *No it doesn't taste the same but*
you learn to get use to it. Especially when you
wanna live. And to answer your other question most
of my people can tell the difference in my food now.
They just mainly come over for conversation, or get
my money.

Danielle: Thank you Mrs. Peterson, I'm
sure your testimony is going to touch the lives in a
lot of households. Have a nice day.

Lillie: *You* too *baby!*

Recipes for Daily Living

Breakfast Ideas:

- turkey bacon (oven cooked), boiled eggs, whole wheat toast

- whole grain waffles with blueberries, freshly squeezed orange juice

- oatmeal with apples, cinnamon sticks, and turkey sausage (light %),

- raisin brain with1/% low-fat milk

- wheat thins with cottage cheese/raspberries

- smoothie breakfast drink: strawberries, ginseng, blueberry, banana, kiwi , grapes (purple), 1 lemon slice, avocado drippings, and 1 carrot

- natural grain pancakes with sugar free syrup, freshly squeezed apple juice

- grits with scrambled eggs, fruit cup

- honey bunches of oats (honey roasted kind) with skim milk

- low-fat cream cheese on green apples, tea with honey and lemon

- cottage cheese with pineapple individually or with rye toast

- baked hash browns and beef jerky well done

- raisins on cantelope, with green tea or 1 glass of concentrated cherry juice

- veggie omelet: tomato, bell pepper, mushroom, shredded low-fat cheese, onion or garlic

(your choice), and 1sprinkle of
Mrs.'s Dash

- 2 apple bran muffins, 1 glass of
fresh fruit juice

Lunch Ideas:

- tuna with rye crackers, celery
sticks, iced tea

- 1 piece of salmon with a toss
salad

- baked potato stuffed with turkey
bits, feta cheese, garlic sprinkles

- baked fish with parsley and red
peppers, homemade lemonade
unsweetened

- low-fat popcorn unbuttered small bag, 1 grapefruit

- **multi mega salad**: green leaf lettuce, cherry tomatoes, peanuts, canola oil or olive oil in place of ranch, raisin, tangerine, radish, oats, baked chicken strips or turkey, black beans, spinach, wheat germ, cashews, broccoli spurs, NO! croutons, and 1 glass of flavored spring water 0% no adding

- 1 rice cake, 1 pomegranate, a healthy soft drink

- corn on the cob (no butter)

  skinless baby shrimps

- peanut butter with apples, potato

  chip crisp (plain no salt or butter)

- homemade chicken soup: carrots,

  boiled chicken, chopped celery,

  Cajun pepper, 1 dash of salt,

  onion powder, boiled potatoes

  (sides) oyster crackers well done

  (darkest selection)

- grilled cheese and tomato soup,

  papaya juice

- **sub sandwich:** whole grain

  bread, roast beef (well done)

mustard, lettuce, tomato, swiss

cheese, lightly spreaded mayo,

banana peppers

Dinner Ideas:

- steamed broccoli and
  cauliflower, baked chicken
  (dark) bran muffins, 1 glass
  of H2O

- catfish baked/coleslaw

- brown rice, smoked turkey,
  peas, lemon water,

- smelts with lima beans

- stuffed peppers with ground
  beef, rice, basil, garlic

powder, tomato sauce,

cottage cheese, corn

- baked sweet potatoes,
  turnip greens, brown pita
  bread

- shredded corn on the cob,
  turkey loaf, banana nut
  bread

- whole grain pasta noodles
  with homemade spaghetti
  sauce

- pinto beans and rice

- beets, liver (baby calf), &
  onion

- squash, chicken breast,
  baby carrots

- lasagna with ground turkey
  or beef, freshly squeezed
  tomatoes for sauce, bell
  pepper, swiss cheese,
  accent seasoning for flavor,
  and 1 glass freshly
  squeezed watermelon juice

- chick peas with cream
  broccoli, choosing to add
  roasted almonds

- brown pasta shell noodles,
  with orange chicken
  drumsticks

- Yeah, Yeah, Yeah, I've heard it all before yuck! But these meals can give you better health.

These recipes were specifically chosen to balance out nutrients, carbohydrates, energy level, proper bowl & urine flow, calcium, iron, vision, cholesterol, oxygen, vitamin C, muscle, bone, etc.

Although, many combinations of fruits and veggies can enhance the well-being of one's health, but choosing the right amount of what the human body needs gives a sure outcome. A satisfying outcome of passing daily body fluids that requires being disposed. Calcium intake for bone density, iron for red blood cells, and oxygen flow.

Healthy food choices also promote weight loss and help maintain a healthy body weight. In contrary to processed foods and sweets which are loaded with calories. Healthy foods are typically low in calorie content despite the fact that they are high in essential nutrients. Thus they enable you to obtain all the nutrients you need without interfering with your weight goals. And by losing excess pounds, you will not only approve your appearance but health too.

Information & Resources

American Cancer Society (cancer.org)

1-877-619-9188

nutritionfacts.org

Personal Knowledge/Education:

UOP, MSU, Grand Valley, U of M

Health and Administration duties

eatright.org (registered dietitians)

www.everydayhealth.com

skincancer.org

cancercenter.com 1-866-512-8502

hopenetwork.org/support

Global Cancer facts & Figures (2nd edition)

Global Cancer Facts & Figures (3rd edition)

cancersupportcommunity.org

Donate Blood: redcross.org

How to reach Danielle:

daniscloset@hotmail.com

Order more copies at lulu.com or

amazon.com

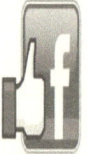 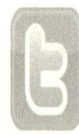 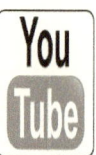

www.ingramcontent.com/pod-product-compliance
Lightning Source LLC
Chambersburg PA
CBHW020405290526
45785CB00005B/2447